E. A. ROBYN

Preparing for the Change of Life

From one girl to another...just some menopause basics and how I'm finding the humor to get through it

Contents

1

Introduction

Let me start off by saying that I have never written a book before, can't say that I ever even thought about doing so either, but I figured since I feel like I might be starting to enter that dreadful stage in my life, very well known to all other women on this planet as menopause, I might as well feel like I'm not doing it alone. That is where you come in. Welcome.

I, like what I would assume is the majority of women, am kind of going into this journey with a little bit of knowledge, a few echoes of other women's complaints and feelings in my head, and a whole lot of hesitation, and for lack of a better way to put it, a blank page.

As a little girl growing up in Texas, all I had as far as family close by were my parents and an older sister (we were not close at all). My parents moved to the small town where I grew up several years before I was born, hours away from any and all other family members. We were out there on our own so to speak. Of course, over time the three (3) of them managed to make a connection to the people that they met in the neighborhood, they met at church, and where they worked, but as a child that was the shyest of the shy, to say the least, that was not the way it was for me. Sure, I knew people, kids on the bus, students and teachers at school, but I was in high school before I began to be comfortable enough to speak to anyone that wasn't in a classroom setting…"Are there any questions boys and girls?"…"no, Ms. Bishop"…you must be crazy if you think I was gonna open up a can of worms by asking any question that I had in front of the whole class. I knew when Ms. Bishop asked, that she was referring to the lesson of that particular day but in my mind I was thinking "Of course I have questions, I have loads of questions, but none that would be appropriate to ask you, my teacher, someone who may or may not blab in the teacher's lounge". You see, it wasn't until later in life that I had enough confidence in myself to broach the subject of anything of a personal nature, and let's face it, it doesn't get any more personal than your monthly cycle. It's horrible enough that you have to endure something like that but to talk about it too? Ugh!!! I think not!!!

Though your mother may warn you of what having a period is like, how it's your path into womanhood, how to get the stains out of your underwear when the pad doesn't stay where you put it (wasn't that the worst?!?!), or how many times to take Midol for the cramps that seem to never get any better despite taking the damn pills, at no time in my life did my mother tell me there was something else to "womanhood". I thought once I got used to having a monthly period that that was all there was to it…NOPE…Girl, I was wrong. The next part, what doctor's tell you is the last part to being a woman, isn't as straightforward as 1) you're gonna have cramps for a couple of days and 2) you're gonna bleed like a stuck pig for the better part of a week. I am finding out that there is more to that "last part" than I thought. I'm taking you with me on the journey to discover the basics of what's considered to be the downfall of every woman's life. Menopause.

INTRODUCTION

We're gonna read about the four (4) different stages of menopause. How they are classically defined, some of the symptoms that you may have to endure along the way, things that are most evidently gonna change, some other conditions or disorders that mimic the same symptoms, the good and the bad of it all. It's probably not gonna be as fun of a reading experience as a romance novel or a great mystery story, but who knows? We may find some humor along the way. Ready or not, here we go...

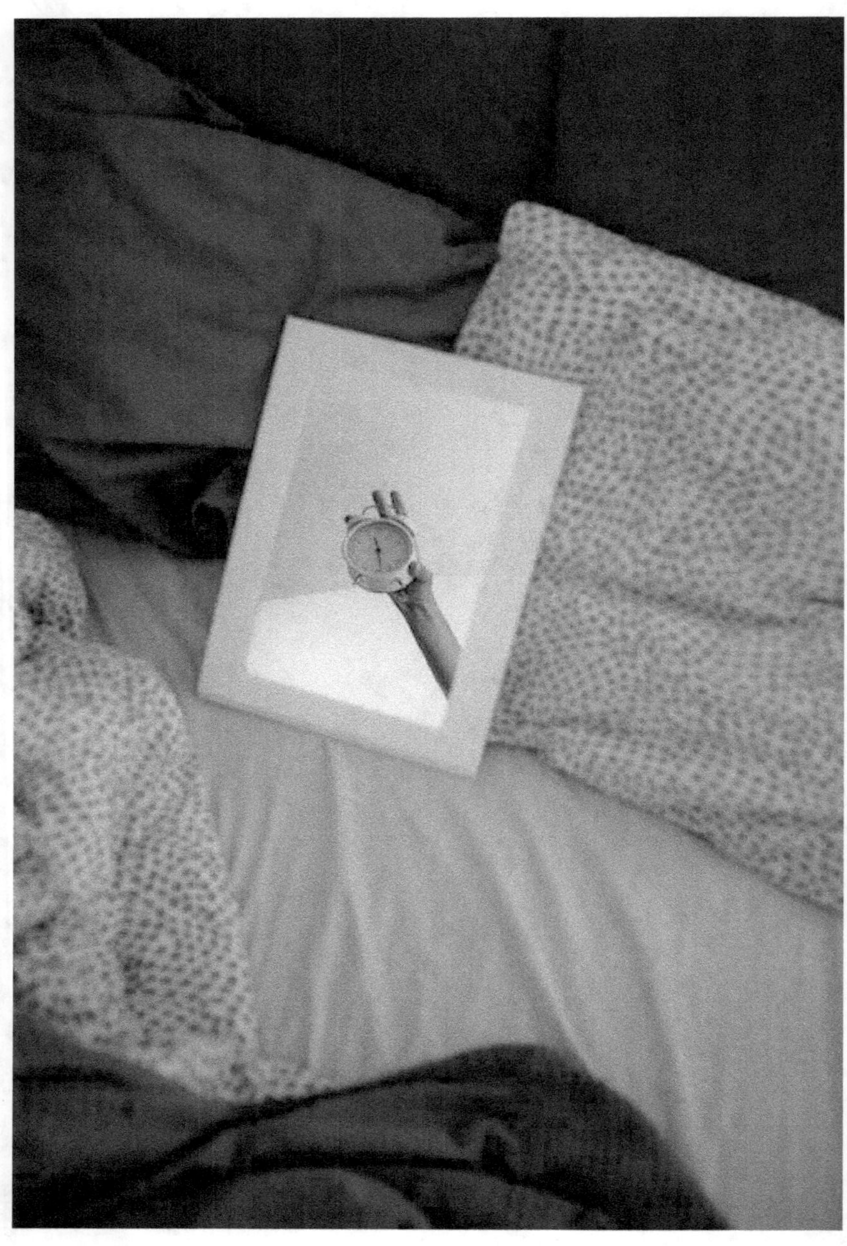

2

The 4 Stages of Menopause

- Premenopause
- Perimenopause
- Menopause
- Postmenopause

So I thought the first place to start was to find out what the 4 stages of menopause were, what I found is as follows:

After exhausting my search through, not one (1) but three (3), different dictionaries, I have come to the conclusion that The American Heritage Dictionary: Based on the New Second College Edition, printed in 1983, Webster's New Dictionary of the English Language, printed in 2006, and The Best Dictionary For Students, printed in 2011, all felt like menopause wasn't worth defining. Can you believe that?? Menopause has been around since way before 1983 so I'm not sure why they didn't feel like they should cover the subject. Hell, at the very least, they could have defined menopause and let us figure the rest out for ourselves, but NO, they didn't do that so I had no choice but to go online and look on Merriam-Webster.com to find some information. This is what I found:

Premenopause- the period of a woman's life that precedes menopause

Perimenopause- the period around the onset of menopause that is often marked by various physical signs

Menopause- the natural cessation of menstruation that usually occurs between the ages of 45 and 55

Postmenopause- having undergone menopause

Does that really help? Or is it just more of the same uncertainty that you already felt? Which is why you started looking for books on the subject in the first place, isn't it? Seems to me like there are actually only two (2) stages to learn about…Pre and Post are pretty self explanatory, "Pre" is before all the fun happens and "Post" is after the party that we wish we didn't have to make an appearance at.

Like I said at the beginning, I am far from a doctor, or a professional of any sort, and I don't want you to think that this is going to be anything more than a collection of information that I managed to gather in my searches of why I felt the way I felt (horrible, sad, hot, and confused). It is merely a faster way for you to gain some insight all in the pages of this one book and not on numerous, time consuming Google searches. What do you say? Should we delve a little deeper?

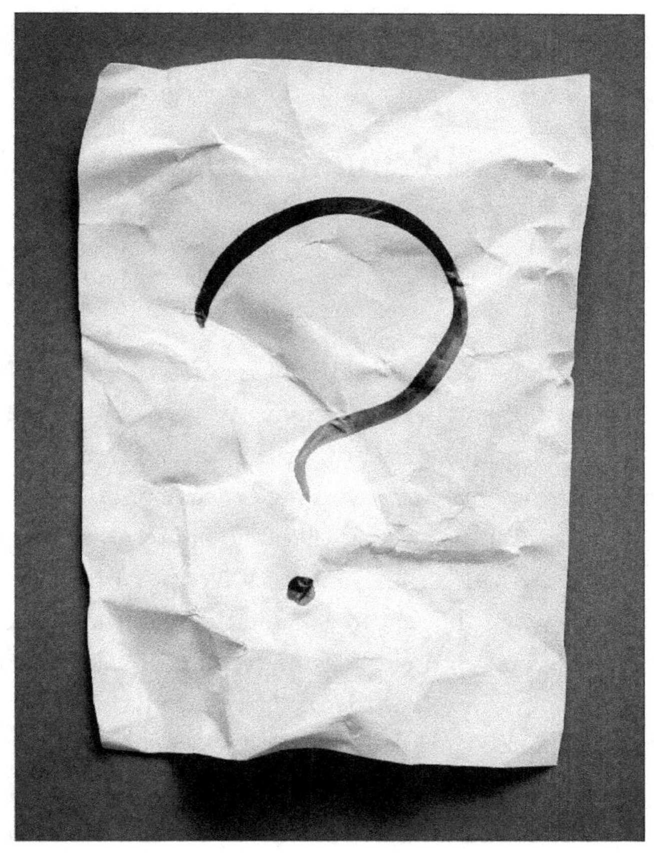

3

Perimenopause

This is the stage that I feel like I am moving into. I just recently turned 45 and have had moments where I wondered if I was headed in that direction or if it was all in my imagination. After one of my yearly exams with my gynecologist at the start of my 40's I asked her if it was possible that I might be entering menopause. She looked at me with a smirk and said "No, you are too young", she didn't ask me why I thought to ask and that was that. After several years of asking and getting the same response I started looking for information and found that the majority of physicians felt like the symptoms stemmed from other things than menopause. It seems to be common that they choose to look in any direction but towards menopause, and I often wondered why.

From what I've read in many different places, perimenopause is the stage before menopause, the period of time that women start to feel differently and notice changes in lots of different areas of her life. This period can last for years and is different for all women. No one's journey is the same as someone else's…Isn't that unfortunate? We may have any or all of the symptoms (I'll cover that in a minute) but I'm sure we'll all agree on something…It's not pleasant! We'd rather be doing something else. Anything else.

Perimenopause is when your menstrual cycles become irregular and some months may pass without having one at all. In most cases the heavy flows that you have experienced all your life get lighter. These two (2) things in particular aren't so bad. By the time you hit your 40's, you've had your period for several decades. DECADES!! Doesn't that make you feel old?? Some of us started before we were teenagers (my sister was ten (10) years old) and some of us were blessed to get this gift of womanhood later in our lives. I, myself, was of the latter group and started at seventeen (17) years old. Think about it, from seventeen (17) years of age to forty five (45) years of age is a total of twenty eight (28) years, with a twenty eight (28) day cycle for that many years…that's approximately three hundred sixty four (364) periods. That's a lot of discomfort, isn't it? What woman isn't excited about not having a menstrual cycle anymore? None that I know.

The cause of your menstrual cycles to be anything but normal is due to hormonal changes in your body, most commonly in your estrogen levels. This is why your periods become irregular and just plain different. It's your body's way of getting you ready to go into menopause. Perimenopause, it's almost like it's holding your hand and walking you to the bus stop. "Go on my dear, you'll be fine".

One of the other things that could happen at this time is pregnancy. Though you aren't as fertile as you were in premenopause, there is still a chance that you could still conceive a child. If that is something that you want, I'm excited for you. If having a baby is the last thing on your mind, may I suggest that you find some sort of protection before you have an oops, but all babies, accidents or not, are gifts from God. You may not have planned it but it was already planned for you.

It is also during this time when you start to see other symptoms (covering those in a minute, remember?) that will have you questioning your sanity. Your hormones are running rampant and with that comes other reasons for you to be uncomfortable.

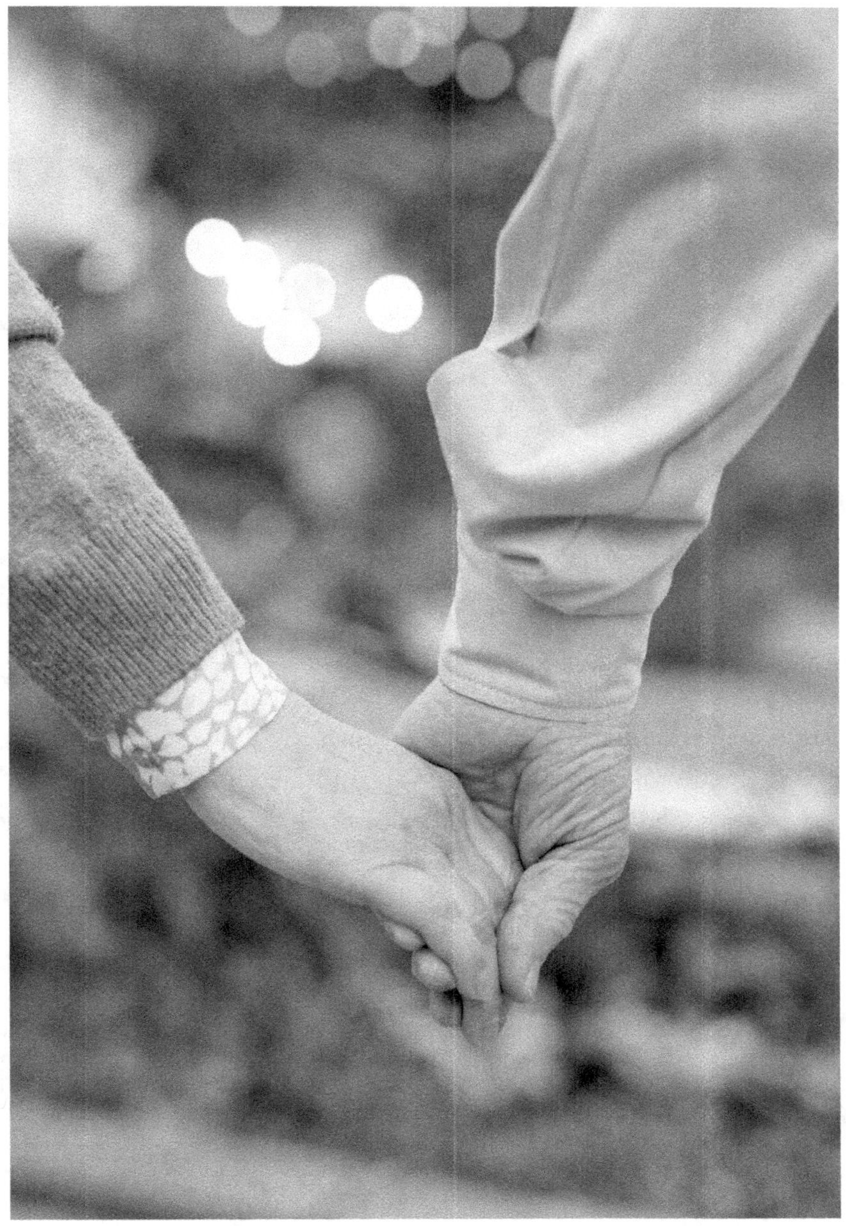

4

Menopause

Menopause is the natural process that a woman's body goes through, most often between forty five (45) years of age and fifty five (55) years of age. It is during this time that her menstrual cycles will diminish in flow and eventually end all together. After going twelve (12) months in a row without having a cycle classifies her as being in the actual stage of menopause. With her cycles ending, it is the end of her reproductive years and therefore the amount of hormones her body is producing has decreased tremendously. Without estrogen and progesterone, you could say that her ovaries are pretty much without a job. They're just there taking up space with nothing to do.

Though the norm is forty five (45) to fifty five (55), it is possible that it can happen earlier than that if the woman has certain medical issues. I have a family member who had cancer at a very young age, was treated with chemotherapy, and went into remission (Thank you, Jesus. God is good!!). Twenty one (21) years later she relapsed in her mid 30's. Her doctors felt like going through chemo again was her best treatment plan, but in doing so, it killed all her reproductive organs and she started showing symptoms of menopause before she was even thirty eight (38) years old. She was prescribed estrogen and progesterone to replace the hormones that her body no longer could produce but it only delayed the inevitable.

Before we go any further, let me just list the symptoms that I found while I was searching:

- Hot flashes
- Mood swings
- Fatigue
- Brain fog
- Overactive bladder
- Incontinence
- Night sweats
- Insomnia
- Weight gain
- Anxiety
- Depression
- Osteoporosis
- Vaginal dryness
- Lack of sex drive

Each of these on their own is bad enough but when you have more than one (1) of them combating you at the same time…you wish you could just pass on this whole section of your life.

5

Hot Flashes

It never fails, when a hot flash comes my way, it happens at the most inopportune time when I can't find a thing to fan myself with, so I start to break out in a sweat, my face gets flushed, and I have a hard time catching my breath. It's not a good time. Not a good time at all!

In an US News article I found online, there are several possible options your doctor might would prescribe you to give you some relief from the dreaded hot flashes

Anti-Depressants
  Paroxetine (brisdelle)
  Venlafaxine (effexor)
  Citalopram (celexa)
  Escitalopram (lexapro)
  Fluoxetine (prozac)
  Paroxetine (paxil)
  Sertraline (zoloft)

Other prescription medications
    Clonidine (catapres)
    Gabapentin (neurontin)
    Pregabalin (lyrica)
    Oxybutynin (ditropan xl or oxytrol)

6

Fatigue & Insomnia

Do you like to sleep? To wake up in the morning feeling well rested? Well that is possibly gonna change. You start to have nights where you toss and turn or don't hardly sleep at all. Insomnia is horrible!!

Fatigue and insomnia are two (2) of the symptoms that confuse me to no end. I have absolutely no energy, I'm so tired from a long day at work, you would think that I could just drift off to sleep with no problem. Wrong! I just lay in bed, staring at the ceiling, yawning and yawning and yawning some more and can not fall asleep to save my soul. If or when I finally do fall asleep, it's not a sound sleep by no means. Awake, asleep, awake, asleep…Not to mention, laying in a puddle because the night sweats are happening so I wake up soaking wet. My clothes, my sheets, my mattress, all soaked. I might as well just get up and change clothes and find a new place to go lay down, trying to make sure it's a wipeable surface because I'll be repeating this process in a little while. How do you get a good night's rest like that? You don't, that's how!

7

Meditation

You can try meditating, some women have found that it is helpful.

Body Scan Meditation - You sit in a quiet place, concentrating on nothing but your breathing and just like the name suggests, you imagine yourself scanning your body from the top to the bottom. Going one part at a time, thinking about what you feel in that particular place. Concentrating on your body will free your mind of everything you were thinking...a mental break from all stress.

Sensory Grounding - You sit with your eyes closed and concentrate on the different sounds around you. Tuning into the rhythm of the sounds around you gives you a break from the sounds in your head allowing you to let go of the tension in your body.

Loving - Kindness Meditation - You sit in a quiet place and think about all the things you like about yourself. Being kind to yourself will help you to feel loved. You can tell everyone around you kind words to make them feel good about themselves, why not yourself?

Bedtime Meditation - After doing your nighttime routine, crawl into bed. Laying very still, breathing in and out very controlled and slow. Don't concentrate on anything but your breathing and let go. Breathe in. Breathe out.

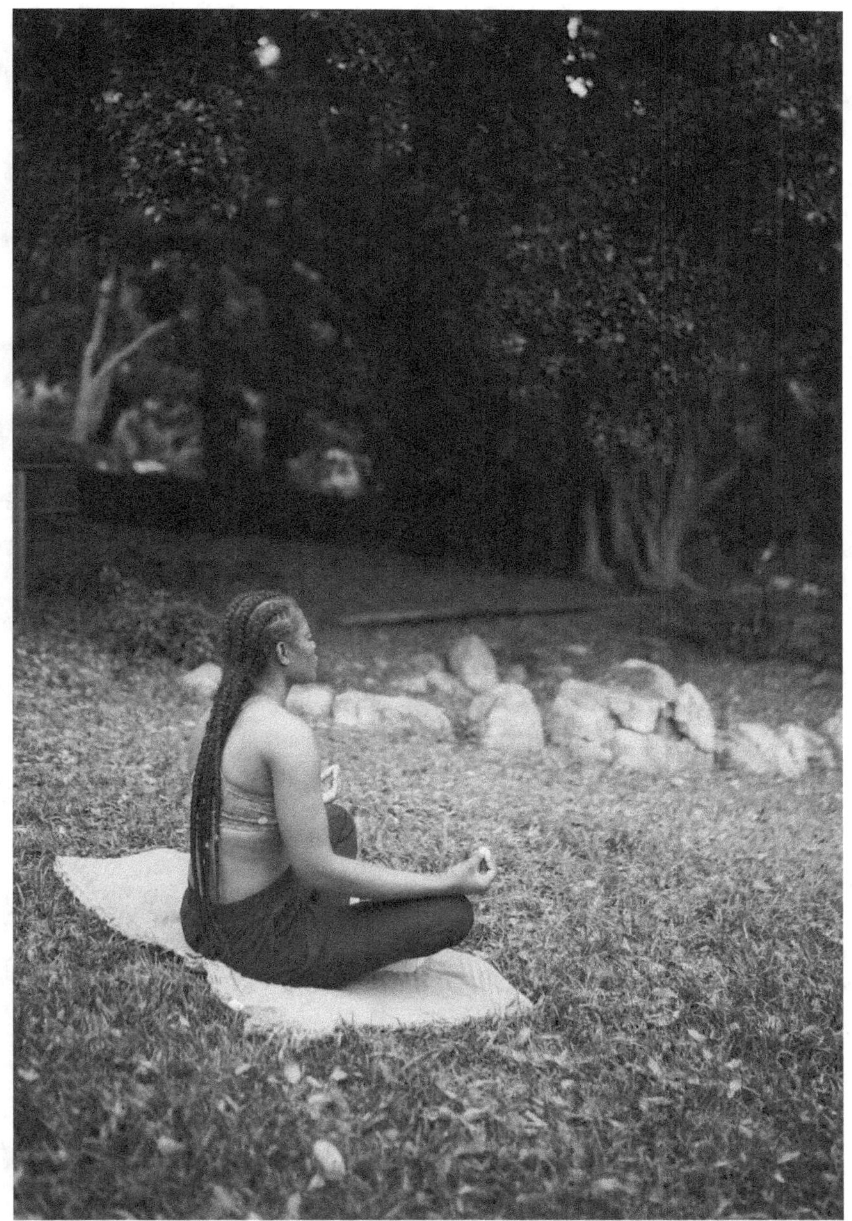

8

Anxiety & Depression

If you have been lucky enough to not have already been diagnosed with anxiety or depression, consider yourself blessed. Some days I do really well and can function like a normal human being flying under everyone's radar and some days it's debilitating and there is no escaping it. Every person I come in contact with on those kinds of days walks on eggshells because my panic attacks are scary for someone who has never experienced them and if it's the depression that's bad that day, I'm a running fountain of tears and they just look at me with a loss of words. To know that there is the slightest chance that both of these symptoms will worsen as I go through menopause scares me to death. How much worse can it get? I'm terrified to find out!!

9

Lack of Sex Drive

I'm not sure how I feel about the lack of sex drive. Is it that you don't want to have sex in general? Or is it the vaginal dryness that makes you not want to do it? There are different brands of lubricant at every drugstore you pass on the street that you could pop in and purchase to help with that problem, but is it just that? Or is it more of what is going through your mind that causes you to not want to have sex? I mean come on, who wouldn't find a sweaty, tired, sad, tearful, and irritable woman sexy? She is every man's dream, isn't she? I know that is what will be going through my mind when that day comes.

10

Overactive Bladder & Incontinence

From what I read, having an overactive bladder isn't because you have menopause per se but more just a contributing factor in general. Due to age and pregnancy, the muscles of a woman's pelvic floor can loosen. This most often will result in the weight of your bladder drooping which in turn causes you to have the need to empty it more often.

You may experience stress induced incontinence, which is when your bladder leaks (a couple of drops at first but overtime can progress to full blown wetting your pants) when you sneeze, cough, laugh, jump, squat, or lift heavy objects. Unless you like that "moist" feeling, you'll need to invest in pantyliners, incontinence pads, diapers, or a pessary. All of those you are probably familiar with except the last one. A pessary is made out of silicone, comes in different shapes and sizes. Your gynecologist has to fit you to determine the proper shape and size you will need to do the trick, as every woman's lady parts are different. It is to be inserted into your vagina for the purpose of holding up the muscles of your pelvic floor to keep your bladder from drooping.

You may also encounter urge incontinence. That's where you all of a sudden feel like you need to urinate but before you know it…it's too late. Yes Ma'am, you're gonna need a change of clothes.

11

Osteoporosis

I'll be honest, I never knew that osteoporosis was a symptom of menopause. Maybe it's like having an overactive bladder and it's not a symptom but just a contributing factor. I always thought it was what my grandma had because she was old, didn't go out in the sun, and didn't like to drink milk. I didn't have a clue that menopause raised a risk for the density of your bones. Who knew? I was today years old when I learned this fact.

I did some digging on the internet and found a list of possible medications you can ask your doctor about in the case you develop osteoporosis.

Estrogen Agonists/ Antagonists
   Raloxifene (evista)

Bisphosphonates
   Alendronate (fosamax)
   Ibandronate (boniva)
   Risedronate (actonel)

Zoledronic Acid (reclast)

12

What Can Be Mistaken For Menopause

Remember when I said that some physicians treat symptoms of menopause as symptoms for other things? Here's a list of some of those things:

- Depression Disorder
- Anxiety Disorder
- Fatigue Syndrome
- Endometriosis
- Polycystic Ovary Syndrome (PCOS)
- Ovarian tumors
- Uterine fibroids
- Angioedema
- Congestive Heart Failure
- Hypothyroidism
- Hyperthyroidism
- Arthritis

All of the above can be very serious and if a patient does have one of these conditions going on with them, they should be treated for that condition in particular. Considering that menopause has similar symptoms, you would think that the doctor would look into the patient's hormone levels before diagnosing her with one of these, then prescribing drugs for that when it wasn't that to begin with. It was menopause and they just assumed otherwise. You went to them for their professional opinion because you didn't feel right and you shouldn't be taking a prescription for some other condition that isn't necessary. How do you feel about this? Am I wrong to feel like this?

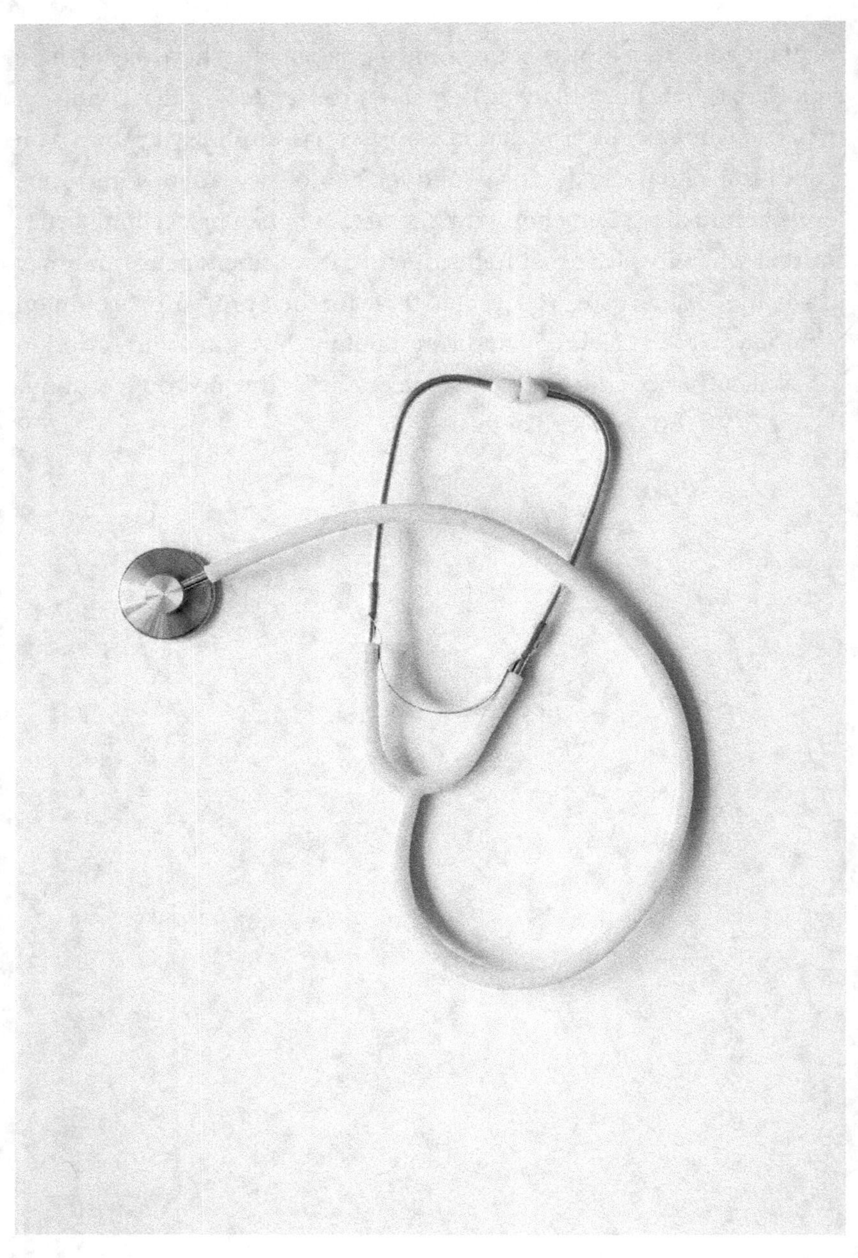

13

Questions To Ask Your Doctors

Maybe you should think about some questions to ask next time you see your physician, whether that visit is with your gynecologist for your annual exam or your primary physician for your yearly wellness visit.

Off the top of my head, here's a few that I came up with:

- Is this menopause or is it something else?
- Is menopause affecting my mental health?
- Is menopause lowering my sex drive or is it something else?
- Is menopause affecting my sleep patterns?
- What can I do for the hot flashes?
- Is there a treatment for vaginal dryness?
- How do I keep my weight from fluctuating?
- What is hormone replacement therapy?
- Will I need hormone replacement therapy?
- Is there anything I can be prescribed to stop some of these symptoms?

- Are the side effects for that prescription worse than the menopause symptoms?
- How do you feel about herbs and supplements? I've read that I could benefit from them.
- How do I do this without losing my sanity in the process?
- How will going through this likely affect my family and friends?

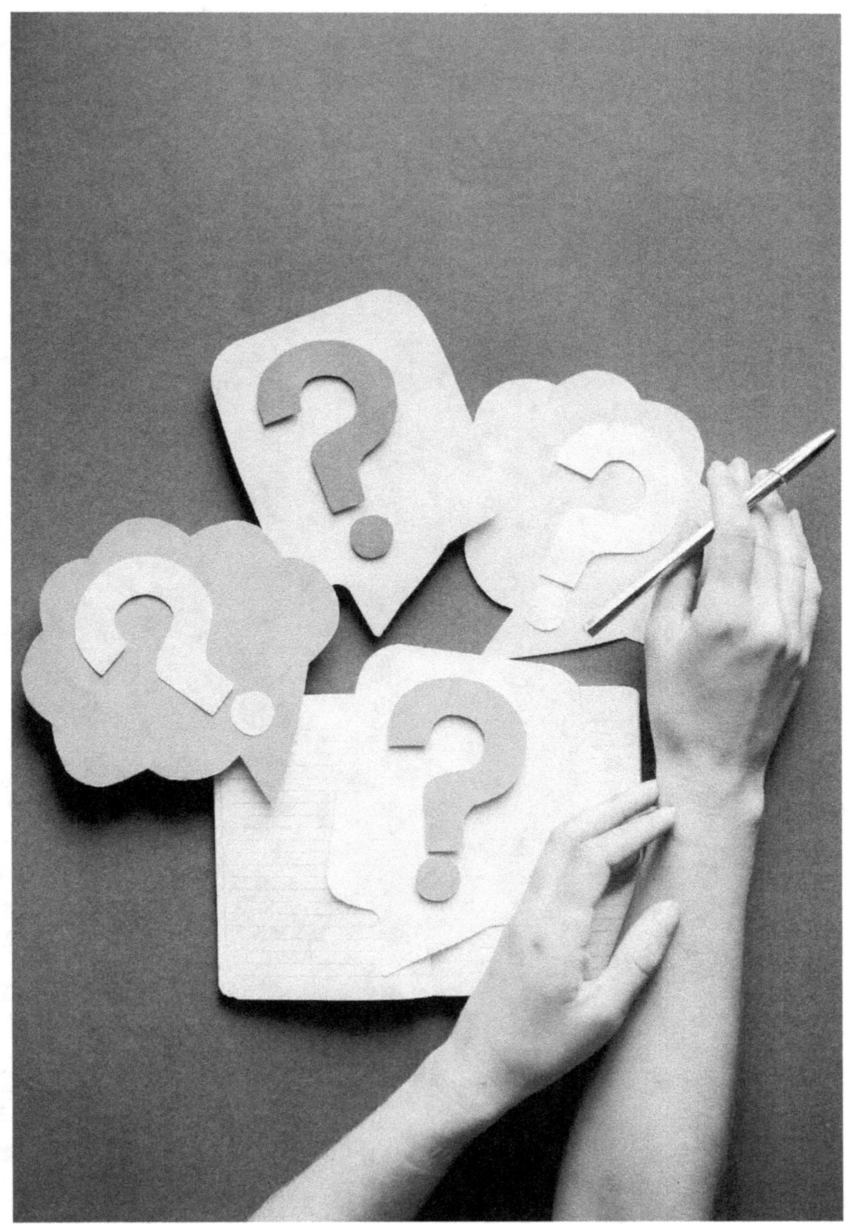

14

Weight Gain

Being a woman in today's world is hard. There are so many different factors that affect your day to day life that for some women, not all women, but some women have trouble controlling their weight. Add in the stress of going through menopause and it amplifies the problem. This is not her fault. She could be putting on weight for several reasons. Two (2) of those reasons are below:

Lower resting metabolic rate

Estrogen levels drop + insulin resistance raises = gradual weight gain

Muscle mass loss

When estrogen levels drop so does muscle mass, low muscle mass can lead to weight gain

I found a list of foods that may help as well:

- Fortified yogurt
- Lean protein

- Salmon
- Spinach
- Almonds
- Quinoa
- Nuts
- Berries
- Leafy green vegetables
- Whole grains
- Turmeric
- Eggs
- Flax seeds

And to repeat my mother, doctor, and every infomercial I've ever seen…

"Drink more water!!!"

15

Herbs & Supplements

On three (3) webpages, I found lists of the different herbs and supplements that will help with all the menopause symptoms. The first one I found was a list of ten (10), second one was a list of twelve (12), and the third was a list of eleven (11). Looking at the lists, some of the herbs and supplements were on all three (3) lists so I felt like though they differed, all the lists were worth mentioning.

Without duplicating the ones that were on all the lists, here's what I found:

- Black cohosh
- Red clover leaf
- Dong quai
- Evening primrose oil
- Maca
- Soy
- Flax seeds
- Ginseng

- Valerian
- Chasteberry
- St . John's wart
- Probiotics
- Apigenin
- Wild yam
- Omega 3 fatty acids
- Calcium
- Vitamin D
- Melatonin
- L-Theanine
- DHEA

16

Don't Feel Like You Are The Only One

You should never feel like you are the only one struggling through this time of your life. There is a whole tribe of us out there going through the same thing. Sure, our symptoms may not be the same or as severe as yours but we're going through it all the same. Even Celebrities can't avoid this part of her life, they suffer too.

Several famous women have spoken on record about their own experiences. Here's a few that I found while doing my research

- Gwyneth Paltrow - on an episode of her Goop Podcast, 2021
- Michelle Obama - on her The Michelle Obama Podcast, 2020
- Oprah Winfrey - in O, The Oprah Magazine, 2019
- Stacy London - wrote on State of Menopause website, unknown
- Cheryl Hines - promotional campaign for AMAG, 2018
- Cynthia Nixon - Stella Magazine, 2017
- Angelina Jolie - Daily Telegraph, 2015

Just knowing that you don't have to go through this alone should make it a little easier to get through. It still won't be easy at times, but it is doable.

17

Just For Laughs

Tampons & pads – "No longer needed, but thank you anyway, I've gone back to wearing diapers."

Hot flashes – "I feel like I'm in a heat wave without a fan. Someone blow on me, I'm hot!!."

Night sweats – "I knew better than to get a spray tan today. My sheets look like they have a silhouette of an Oompa-Loompa right where I was laying."

Mood swings – "One minute I'm sweet as an angel, and the next thing I know, the Wicked Witch of the West has rode in on her broom."

Brain fog – "I used to walk around with my head in the clouds, now I think it's more like smog."

Emotions – "Nowadays, I cry at the drop of a hat, over the stupidest thing, I thought that ended with being pregnant."

Bathroom breaks – "I'm trying to decide on a new wallpaper for my bathroom at home so I have to go take a peek in every restroom we pass. Hold my purse, I'll be right back."

Vaginal dryness – "With all the sweating I do, why is my vagina the only thing on my body that is dry?

BTW – isn't By the way, it's Bring the wine

WTF – isn't What the f***?!?!, it's Where's the fan?!?!

IRL – isn't In real life, it's I require lube

HBD – isn't Happy Birthday, it's Having bad day

FBO – isn't Facebook official, it's Forget being optimistic

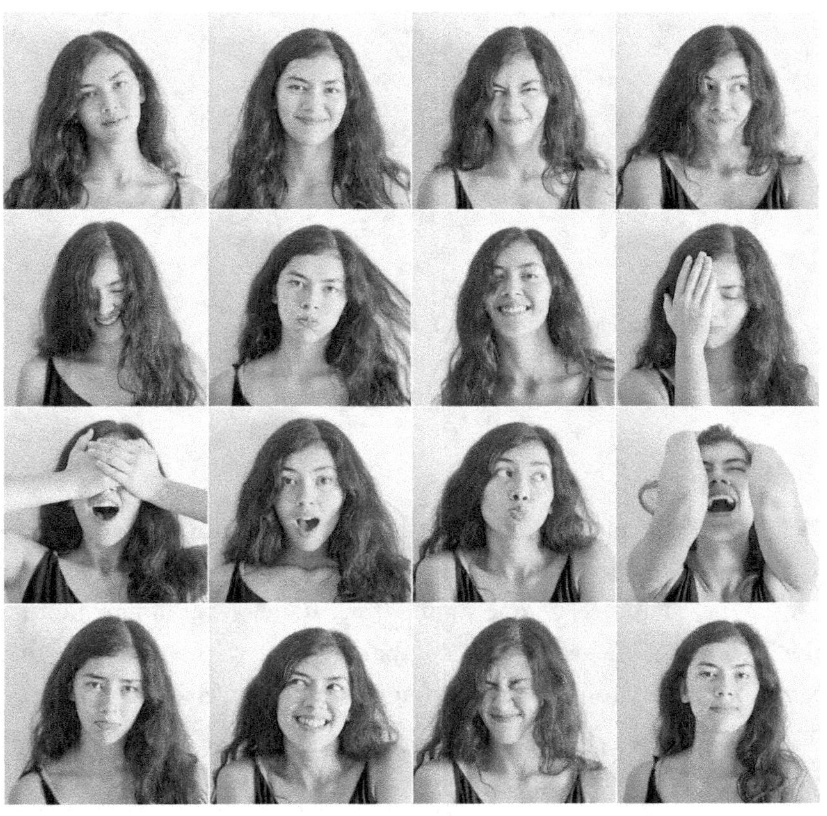

18

Conclusion

If you have made it to this page, I want to thank you for taking the time to go along on my journey. No one likes to travel alone, therefore, no one should learn alone. What did my mother always tell me?…Misery loves company…Who wants to go through bad experiences alone? Not me. If not for anything else, just for moral support.

I know what you are probably thinking…She could have gone more in depth on things…I most certainly could have but then I risked you getting bored and closing the book like most kids do in school when they get tired of hearing the same lesson day after day.

Could some of the facts I found and wrote about be off some? Maybe not as verbatim as a medical journal? Sure, I told you in the beginning that I wasn't a professional and I continue to stand behind that. I am nothing more than a girl who thinks she may be starting to experience menopause. What no one ever mentioned to me as a child but now refers to it as "an absolute nightmare". Gee thanks family and friends. Way to go to leave a girl hanging. That's ok though. I am tough. I am resilient. I am a warrior. I am enough.

I don't know you in person but feel like we share a common bond so I want you to know that those things apply to you as well. You are tough. You are resilient. You are a warrior. You are enough.

If you found the pages of this book even the least bit helpful, be it to learn new facts, or just to give you something to smile about today, then my job here is done. I finished what I set out to do. All I ask of you now, is to go to Amazon, find this book, and leave a positive review. Feel free to recommend it to your friends and ask them to leave a positive review as well. It would be most appreciated.

May your menopause journey be a good one, my friend.

Always remember to take care of yourself so that you are around to take care of others.

Smile and find your happy place.

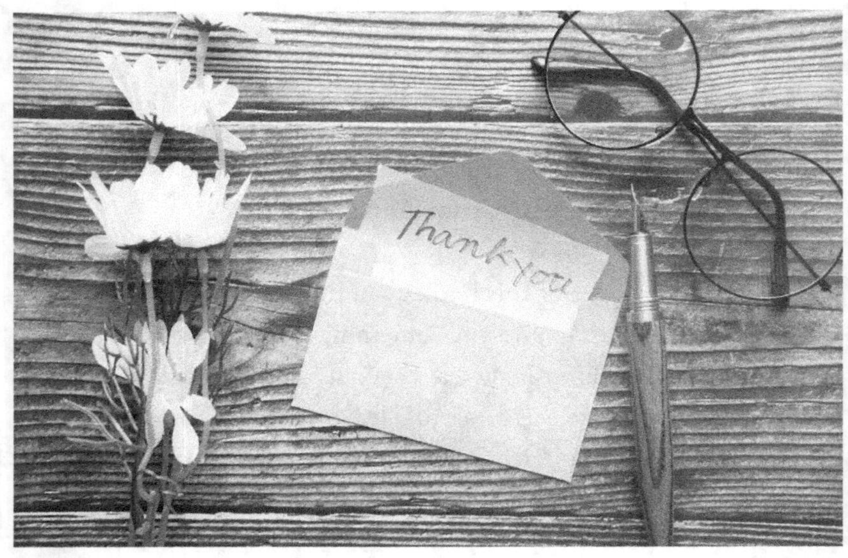

19

Resources

Merriam Webster Incorporated. (2023). *definition.* Merrian-Webster. Retrieved November 5, 2023, from https://www.merriam-webster.com/

Professional, C. C. M. (2021). *Menopause.* Cleveland Clinic. Retrieved November 6, 2023, from https://my.clevelandclinic.org/health/diseases/21841-menopause

Fulton, A. (2022, July 5). *Is It Menopause or Something Else?* HealthyWomen. Retrieved November 6, 2023, from https://www.healthywomen.org/your-health/is-it-menopause-or-something-else

Health Content Provider. (2005, November). Conditions with Similar Symptoms as: Menopause | Complementary and Alternative Medicine | St. Luke's Hospital. *St Luke's Hospital.* Retrieved November 7, 2023, from https://www.stlukes-stl.com/health-content/medicine/33/000470.htm

Watson, S. (2023, March). *Symptoms of Menopause from Ages 40 to 65.* Healthline. Retrieved November 9, 2023, from https://www.healthline.com/health/menopause/symptoms-of-menopause#Ages-50-to-55

Ld, A. H. R. (2020, September). *10 Herbs and Supplements for Menopause.* Healthline. Retrieved November 10, 2023, from https://www.healthline.com/nutrition/menopause-herbs

Rowe, MD, N. (2023, September). *The Most Popular Supplements for Menopause (and Which Ones Really Work).* GoodRx Health. Retrieved November 10, 2023, from https://www.goodrx.com/conditions/menopause/supplements

Johnson, MD, T. (2022, November). *11 Supplements for Menopause Symptoms.* WebMD. Retrieved November 10, 2023, from https://www.webmd.com/menopause/ss/slideshow-menopause

Upham, B. (2023, June). *Healthy Foods for Menopause.* Everyday-Health.com. Retrieved November 10, 2023, from https://www.everydayhealth.com/menopause/healthy-foods-to-eat-during-menopause/

Momaya, A. (2022, October). *10 Best Foods To Eat During Menopause - HealthifyMe.* HealthifyMe. Retrieved November 10, 2023, from https://www.healthifyme.com/blog/best-foods-to-eat-during-menopause/

The Best Exercises to Help You Lose Weight During Menopause. (2021, March). Evernow. Retrieved November 10, 2023, from https://w

ww.evernow.com/learn/the-best-exercises-to-help-you-lose-weight-during-menopause

Goldwert, L. (2022, November). *Meditation Techniques to Help with Menopause Symptoms*. Stripes. Retrieved November 10, 2023, from https://iamstripes.com/blogs/mental-health/meditation-techniques-to-help-with-menopause-symptoms

HealthDay. (2023, June). *The Most Common Menopause Medications, Explained*. US News & World Report. Retrieved November 10, 2023, from https://www.usnews.com/news/health-news/articles/2023-06-20/the-most-common-menopause-medications-explained

What to Know About Menopause Medications. (2023, May). Retrieved November 10, 2023, from https://www.healthcentral.com/condition/menopause/menopause-drugs-medications

7 Celebrities Who Have Talked Openly About Menopause. (2022, March). Retrieved November 10, 2023, from https://www.healthcentral.com/condition/menopause/celebrities-menopause

Does Menopause Cause Urinary Incontinence? (2020, August). Dedicated to Women. Retrieved November 10, 2023, from https://dedicatedtowomenobgyn.com/posts/does-menopause-cause-urinary-incontinence/#:~:text=This%20loss%20of%20bladder%20control,likely%20to%20have%20urinary%20incontinence.

www.ingramcontent.com/pod-product-compliance
Lightning Source LLC
Chambersburg PA
CBHW071128260726

48661CB00006B/2717